Winning the Fight Against Sepsis

What Every Nurse Should Know

Melissa Moye

First published by Dog Ear Publishing
4010 W. 86th Street, Ste H
Indianapolis, IN 46268
www.dogearpublishing.net

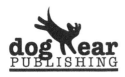

ISBN: 978-1-4575-1368-8

This book is printed on acid-free paper.

Printed in the United States of America

AUTHOR'S NOTE

I love to write. I've written two fiction novels, one that I'm self-publishing (the first in a paranormal series about a traveling nurse, *The Traveler: In the Beginning*, available at Amazon and Barnes and Noble), a screenplay, numerous short articles for nursing magazines, and now this educational booklet on sepsis.

I would like to thank Connie Wood, RN, Critical Care Educator, for suggesting this topic to me when I said I wanted to write a nonfiction book for nurses. I would also like to thank my director, Cindy Keller, RN, for her support and contact information.

Thanks especially to my husband, Bill, for his endless hours of love and encouragement and for never complaining of my hours at my computer.

I dedicate this book to my dad, who died of cardiopulmonary failure secondary to sepsis in 2008.

TABLE OF CONTENTS

CHAPTER 1

Introduction to Sepsis

SOME OF THE EARLIEST EVIDENCE of wound management dates back to 10,000 BCE. Skulls have been found from that time with evidence of scrapings and scratches from their healers' attempts at treatment.

Man has fought sepsis since ancient times. In the fourth century BC, Hippocrates mentioned that "humors" and "foul vapors" cause disease, and he gave instructions regarding dry wound therapy. We find evidence of man's attempt to treat sepsis in Mesopotamia, Egypt, Greece, and everywhere else throughout the ancient world. Numerous written records such as the Eber's Papyrus in Egypt have been found describing such medical treatments.

Bacteria, fungus, viruses, and parasites constitute thousands of pathogens that commonly cause sepsis. They are found everywhere in our environment. Some organisms, such as yeast in bread, are harmless and can be beneficial, but many can cause us to become very ill. They can originate from almost anywhere on or inside our bodies, usually from local infections. The most common areas for local infections to occur include the lungs, abdomen, urinary tract, skin, bones, and central nervous system. If left untreated in a healthy patient or occurring in an immune-compromised patient, these organisms can cause a systemic reaction known as sepsis.

New strains of bacteria such as VRE (Vancomycin-resistant enterococcus) and MRSA (Methicillin-resistant staphylococcus aureus) are becoming more difficult to treat, as they have mutated and become resistant to antibiotics. These genetic mutations are known as superbugs.

Certain obvious signs and symptoms are exhibited as sepsis begins, including fever, increased breathing rate, and rapid heart rate. If a patient displays these symptoms, immediate blood work should be done. Results indicative of sepsis include an elevated or decreased white blood cell count, elevated plasma lactate levels, worsening kidney function, and more.

The body goes through a cascade of events as it fights sepsis. It begins with an inflammatory reaction to bacterial or other toxins, followed by altered blood clotting and, finally, organ death as the immune system is pushed into overdrive. Survival depends on immediate and accurate treatment.

This book focuses on the early identification of sepsis and on the immediate actions that a nurse should take when symptoms indicate that a patient is becoming septic. Treatments suggested herein are taken from the global Surviving Sepsis Campaign developed by the European Society of Critical Care Medicine, the International Sepsis Forum, and the Society of Critical Care Medicine to form guidelines for the treatment of sepsis.

Sepsis affects an estimated 750,000 people a year (Goldberg, 2011), adds 8 million days in the hospital, and costs more than 20 billion dollars to our nation's annual healthcare cost (Hughes, 2011). With the advancing age, increased obesity, and worsening health of our population, we must have nurses educated in specific sepsis protocols.

Successfully defeating sepsis depends on first identifying the septic patient by his or her signs and symptoms; next obtaining lab test results such as blood cultures, kidney function, lactate levels, and a complete cell count to confirm a diagnosis of sepsis; and finally initiating the sepsis bundle protocols.

References

1. Goldberg, Carey. (2011, February 28). With Sepsis, Higher Cost May Not Mean Living Longer. *Common Health Reform and Reality.*_WBUR.org Boston. Retrieved from http://commonhealth.wbur.org/ 2011/02/with-sepsis-higher-cost-may-not-mean-living-longer/

2. Hughes, James M. (2011, March 9). Preserving the Lifesaving Power of Antimicrobial Agents. *JAMA.* 305, (10), 1027 Retrieved from http://jama.amaassn. org/content/early/2011/02/21/jama.2011.279.full

CHAPTER 2

The History of Sepsis

SEPSIS OCCURS WHEN AN INVADING organism is introduced into the bloodstream. Sepsis can originate from any source such as a wound, the urinary tract, the lungs, bones, the abdomen, the brain, or an intravenous catheter. If left untreated, sepsis initiates a cascade of events that may result in septic shock and death.

Sepsis is not a new disease process known only to our era. It has been mentioned frequently throughout history by many ancient scholars. In fact, Homer was the first person to mention sepsis in a medical context more than 2700 years ago. Some of the earliest civilizations such as those in Mesopotamia, Arabia, Egypt, and Greece left record of their medical practices in the form of clay tablets, the Sanskrit documents (2000 BCE), the Smith Papyrus (1650 BCE), and the Ebers Papyrus (1550 BCE).

The Ebers Papyrus was written in Thebes, Egypt around 1550 BCE. It contains notes from at least 40 sources and lists 876 remedies, pharmacopoeia, and doctors' medicinal formulae. It lists the symptoms, diagnosis, treatment, and prescriptions for many diseases and injuries, along with the suggested prayers and incantations for them. It specifically mentions garlic as being used in the treatment of wounds.

One of the earliest known treatments for wounds comes from Egypt in 1550 BCE and involves the preparation of an ointment of lard, honey, and lint applied directly to the wound. Honey kills bacteria by pulling the water out of it and converts the oxygen and glucose into a form like hydrogen peroxide, a potent disinfectant used worldwide today.

The ancient Egyptians used other antibacterial substances, as well:

- frankincense and myrrh—fragrant resins that preserve human remains
- onions and garlic—plants that contain a powerful antibiotic called allicin
- radishes—roots that contain raphanin, another powerful antibiotic source

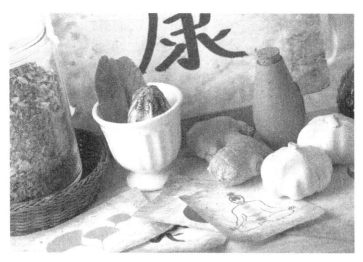

Alternative therapy.

Other Egyptian wound therapies resemble current modalities. They used a moist wound-healing technique in which a wound was closed via suturing or, in a diseased wound, debridement was followed by antibacterial therapy. (It is unknown whether the antibacterial therapy was intentional or not.) They used wine, vinegar, and hot water to cleanse wounds, and then they used a dry powder mixture of different metals (mercury, zinc, silver, and copper) to prevent inflammation. They would use strips of linen that had been soaked in honey, oil, and lint to pack wounds.

It is now known that the mixture of copper and wine created a strong antibacterial compound that we now call copper acetate and that the packed wound created an oxygen-poor environment that stimulated angiogenesis (the growth of new capillary blood vessels that help with healing). Furthermore, the combination of products the ancient Egyptians used in bandages prevented the linen from sticking to the wound and resulted in a nonadherent type of dressing. It is similar to what we currently use today.

The ancients used silver in plasters to cover open wounds and also to purify the drinking water of their monarchs.

Ancient Sumerian texts outline Sumerian wound care management: "Cleanse the wound with beer, then bandage with a cloth soaked in wine and turpentine." (Miller, 2005). Current research has revealed that the antiseptic properties of wine are due to the high number of polyphenols it contains.

In the years 460–370 BCE, Hippocrates stated that pus was not a natural component in the healing process. His advice was similar to that of the Sumerians: "Cleanse the wound with wine, apply a bandage, and then pour wine on the bandage." (Miller, 2005). Hippocrates believed in first carefully monitoring the patient, and he advocated a dry wound therapy by the use of the recuperative powers of nature.

Infected wounds have often been treated with wine and vinegar since the age of Hippocrates. It was originally believed that the alcohol content of wine served as an antibiotic source, but recent chemical analysis has found the antibiotic properties to be due to a substance called malvoside. The acid content of vinegar is another powerful antiseptic that kills the germs that cause disease.

During the time of Hippocrates, sepsis was viewed as a process of dangerous, odorous, biologic decay or putrefaction. The ancient Greeks believed this process occurred within the body as a result of biological breakdown and that autointoxication was a result of these dangerous principles. Aristotle, and later the Romans, proposed that sepsis resulted from the production of invisible living creatures that lived in the putrid fumes (named miasmata) within swamps. Early public health initiatives in Roman cities were geared toward fighting the spontaneous generation of tiny dangerous animals by eliminating those perceived deadly swamps.

Because many medications and antibiotics had not been discovered yet, ancient peoples used a variety of plants for their herbal medicinal properties. In 2735 BCE, Sheng Nung, a Chinese emperor, wrote about fever and how to treat it with herbal medicine. Sheng Nung was known as the Divine Plowman and is considered the father of Chinese agriculture. He experimented with the healing properties of plants, and *The Herbal Classic of the Divine Plowman* is the result of his years of work. It mentions more than 150 illnesses that can be treated with herbs and lists more than 250 herbs by taste, function, and health benefit.

The first science-based medical manuscript, titled *De Medicina*, was written by Aulus Cornelius Celsus sometime

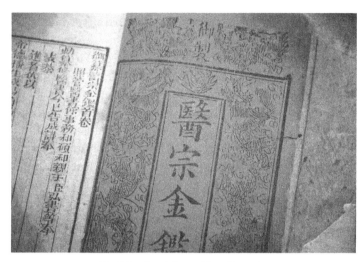

Medicine book from Qing Dynasty.

between the years 25 BCE and 50 CE. In it are described the four cardinal signs of infection that we still use to this day: rubor (redness), calor (warmth), dolor (pain), and tumor (swelling). Celsus also mentions the importance of thorough wound cleansing: "Clean the wound of old blood because this can cause infection and change into pus, which inhibits wound healing." (Moüs, Heule, Legerstee, and Steven, 2009).

Claudius Galen (130–200 CE), a physician to the gladi- ators, agreed with Hippocrates's practice of medicine. He performed many experiments and was a proponent for questioning established doctrines to expand scientific knowledge. One of his theories that proved to be terribly wrong was that pus was essential for healing. His works were translated into many languages, and they continued to be the unofficial guide for the medical treatment of wounds for more than 15 centuries, until our modern era.

The Dark Ages arrived with the fall of the Roman Empire around the year 410 CE. The years that followed were barbaric, and people lived in misery and filth. Diseases such as smallpox and measles became epidemic as they were spread via the trade routes that had previously carried supplies and wealth. The plague arrived in the year 542 CE on rats that stowed away on ships from distant lands. Half of the world's population died, and there was no one left to work on farms or to feed the survivors.

The plague actually had three major outbreaks that resulted in millions of deaths worldwide. The first was the plague of Justonian in the 6th century CE. Then came the Black Death in the 14th century and, finally, the bubonic plague in 1665–1666.

There was an almost total lack of scientific or medical advancement during the Dark and Middle Ages. Unhealthy sanitation, poor hygiene, endemic diseases, dirt, filth, and poor diets kept the average life spans at that time to less than twenty years. Surviving just to the age of five was considered a miracle.

There were no hospitals where educated physicians could give care to the sick and wounded. In fact, no educated person would touch a sick patient at that time, as sick people were considered to be unclean. It was a time when the Church ruled the world and when people believed in magic and other supernatural solutions to their illnesses. Disease was thought to be the result of sin and vice, not of poor hygiene or other natural causes.

After the fall of Rome in the 5th century, in the Islamic empire, knowledge of medicine flourished. It was strongly influenced by Greek medicine and by astrologic teachings from Asia and Egypt. The Islamic civilization established several hospitals, such as one in Damascus in the year 1160 and the Al-Mansur Hospital in Cairo in 1276. Al-Mansur was the first hospital that emphasized science, teaching, and social service. It was one of Islam's great physicians, Rhazes (860–930 CE) who distinguished smallpox from measles.

Scientific advancement suffered in Europe under the control of the Church. Christian theology focused its attention on curing the soul rather than the body, and the Church lost its power as people realized it was not curing their illnesses or solving their problems. As those dark ages were left behind, a new age of enlightenment called the Renaissance began. The Renaissance was a time when the Church lost authority and when some of the beliefs of the ancients returned.

The Renaissance began in Italy in the 1300s and spread first throughout Northern Europe. People began to get more interested in the arts and sciences, which led to a revival of classical learning, art, and architecture. This was a time of great growth and advancement in science and medicine.

Prior to the Renaissance, the care of the sick and injured had been given to the Church. Dark Age Christian hospitals, located in monasteries, were run mostly by untrained nuns and monks who used simple foods, herbs, and the washing of wounds as their treatment. The majority of European hospitals up to this point had been nothing but alms houses, places for the poor, sick, and elderly. One of the first examples of a hospital in Western Europe was at the monastery of St. Gaul, where, in 820 CE, it had rooms for six patients, a medical herb garden, a pharmacy, and a special area for the lodging of a physician.

For hundreds of years in the Dark Ages, the Church had done nothing to advance medicine. The Church slowly lost its control of medicine. By the year 1130, monks and clerics were forbade to practice medicine, and the Church had stopped providing care to the sick.

In Europe, as more and more hospitals were being created, the laws that governed physicians' education became stricter. In the year 1140, the king of Sicily ruled that no one could practice medicine without a degree from a university.

From the 12th to the 17th centuries, Western Europe was plagued by almost continuous wars. There were many and varied battlefield injuries that required special treatment. The injured were cared for either by their comrades in arms or by women camp-followers until the field hospital was introduced in the 16th century. Serious injuries were attended to by barber-surgeons, or field cutters who were paid a high bounty and employed by the army commander. This led to the formation of a new kind of wound surgeon highly skilled in caring for wounded soldiers as these surgeons learned their trade in the battlefield.

Ambroise Paré was an inexperienced barber-surgeon who published some experiences in 1545. He stated that he dressed many wounds with egg yolk, rose oil, and turpentine after he ran out of his boiling oil. He found that when the next morning arrived, wounds treated with the boiling oil were in much worse condition and the men had more fever and pain than those treated with his new egg remedy.

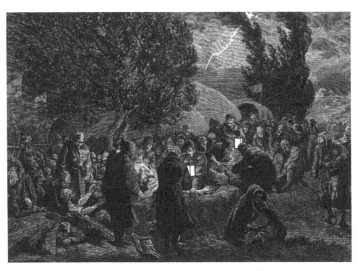

Doctors working in battlefield. Appeared in the *Illustrated London News* Saturday, October 20, 1877.

The Renaissance was a time of great growth both in medical and scientific terms. Many of the previously heinous and barbaric treatments were abandoned, and new, more humane, therapies were adopted (such as the egg yolk, rose oil, and turpentine mentioned above). More and more new discoveries were made in the 1800s, as people no longer feared religious persecution for going against the Church.

The microscope was one of the greatest inventions of the scientific and medical community. It allowed a world of previously unknown living organisms to be seen and studied, and it changed the course of human history. It's hard to say exactly who invented the microscope, or when it was invented. One of the first references made about glass and crystal was during the time of Pliny the Elder in the first century CE, but it was Euclid who wrote about the rules of reflected light in the third century BCE and who is considered to be the father of optics.

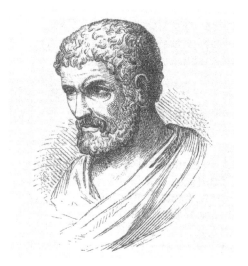

Euclid.

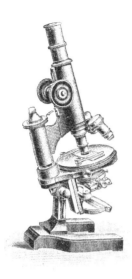

Microscope.

Robert Hooke was the first person to mention seeing microbes under a microscope, in the year 1665. He reported that he could see and identify the cellular structure of plants.

The first person to describe bacteria was Anton Van Leeuwenhoek in 1668. He developed the skill of lens grinding after he traveled to England and saw drawings of magnifications of cloth. He made many different microscopes out of items such as gold and silver. He viewed a variety of substances such as his semen and the scum from his own teeth, and he was able to identify microbes such as protozoa and microscopic algae. Even though he reported his findings to the Royal Society of London in 1676, two hundred years passed before the science of microbiology began to flourish.

By the 1900s, hospitals were becoming more common, not only for the sick and injured but also as centers of education and research. Change was still hard to accept, however, and often, the doctors were ridiculed and suffered personal harassment for their ideas.

For instance, in 1841, a young doctor named Ignaz Semmelweis was hired to run a maternity ward in Vienna. He noted that mothers' deaths from puerperal sepsis (child bed fever) was 18% higher for the patients who were treated by physicians than those treated by the midwives. He was fired when he suggested that the physicians must be contributing to this somehow.

Semmelweis got a new job, and after one of his friends cut himself during an autopsy and died, Semmelweis reasoned that some kind of an invisible agent had caused the deaths of his friend and the mothers. He believed that this invisible agent was transferred from the autopsy room to the birthing room and that the physicians were infecting the mothers with their dirty lab coats. He made a rule that the doctors would change their lab coats and wash their hands in a disinfectant before they examined patients or assisted with births. The death rate dropped by 2/3 in the hospital, but Semmelweis was fired again for his offensive ideas. This happened a few more times before the poor man died years later of what looked to be puerperal sepsis in an insane asylum.

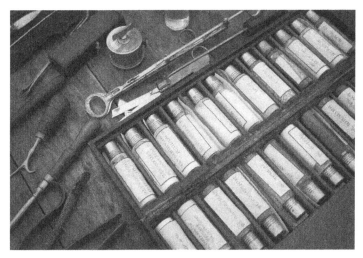

Old-fashioned medical supplies

In 1842, Oliver Wendell Holmes of Harvard also recommended that doctors wash their hands when they went to the wards from the autopsy rooms. He specifically advised that they wash with a calcium chloride solution to prevent the spread of infection. (Miller, 2005) Though time has proved that both Semmelweis and Holmes were correct in their views, neither of them received a warm welcome from the medical community for their suggestions.

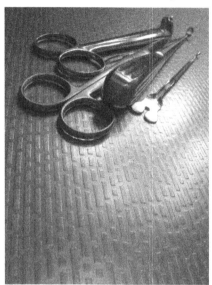

Old surgical instruments.

Operations in the 19th century were performed under the worst conditions possible. Medical instruments weren't clean, as they often were simply wiped with a cloth or sharpened on the surgeon's boot between uses. Floors of operating rooms were not clean and were often covered in blood, pus, and feces. Consequently, 80% of patients developed hospital gangrene, with a nearly 50% rate of mortality. Because of the stench from all the dead bodies and the resulting "bad air," some people believed that the infections came about as a result of spontaneous generation.

Louis Pasteur is known as one of the greatest benefactors to humanity. He was born in France in 1822 and used his knowledge as a chemist to become the founder of microbiology. He proved that the theory of spontaneous generation was wrong, and through systematic observation and experiments, he proved that fermentation, putrefaction, and disease were caused by living microbes. He was able to put an end to the centuries of ignorance and superstitions that had long held back the progress of medicine.

Pasteur discovered that many plant and animal diseases were caused by yeasts and bacteria. In 1885, he formulated the fundamental principles of the germ theory of disease, which resulted in improved sanitation, disinfection, and the use of antibiotics. He discovered the process of pasteurization that has resulted in safe food and milk production, and he discovered better methods of producing chemicals and drugs that resulted in increased agricultural production. Perhaps his most important work, saving more lives than any other medical advancement, is the process of immunization.

Following in Pasteur's footsteps, Robert Koch also had an enormous influence on the science of bacteriology. Through his research on organisms such as anthrax and tuberculosis, Koch discovered a procedure that can prove whether an organism is the cause of a disease. This process is known as Koch's Postulates, and it consists of the following four steps:

1. Isolate the suspected agent from a diseased victim.
2. Grow the agent in a pure culture.
3. Infect a healthy host to prove that the organism is what produced the disease.
4. Isolate the same organism from the new victim. (Hurlbert, 1999)

In the years that followed the formation of Koch's Postulate, many discoveries were made about the relationship between bacteria and yeasts and their different disease processes. Once this link was formed, it wasn't long before the age of antisepsis began.

Antiseptics may be considered as a precursor to antibiotics. The first person to link the suppuration of wounds with Louis Pasteur's discovery of the fermentation process was Joseph Lister. He published a paper in April 1867 on antisepsis that stated, "All the local inflammatory mischief and general febrile disturbance which follow severe injuries are due to the irritation and poisonous influence of decomposing blood or sloughs." (Miller, 2005)

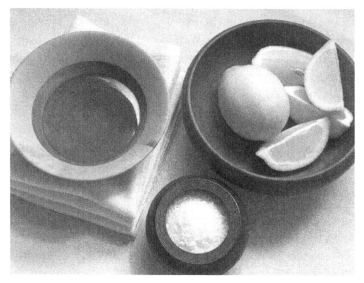

Lemons, honey, and salt are well-known for their antiseptic and medicinal properties.

Lister achieved better wound healing, fewer amputations, and an improved mortality rate (dropping from 45% to 15%) after he began to apply carbolic acid to wounds. He also began to sterilize his medical instruments and bandages with phenol solutions, but other physicians did not follow his example because no one had yet to link microorganisms with the development of sepsis. Full-strength phenol was being used in patients who developed gangrene from severe infections, while another popular antiseptic, hydrogen peroxide, was in decline because of reports of air emboli formation in patients.

While searching for a better antimicrobial agent, Fleming discovered lysozyme in 1921. It is a naturally occurring substance found in egg whites, milk, pus, saliva, tears, and white blood cells that dissolves and digests bacteria. It was found to be a key component in the body's immune defense system.

As important as the discovery of lysozyme was in the fight against microorganisms, Fleming's next discovery created the first real breakthrough in the search for ways to fight infections. After serving as a captain in World War I and working in battlefield hospitals in France, he was elected Professor of Bacteriology at St. Mary's School in 1928. In the same year, while experimenting with an influenza virus, he discovered penicillin, which is effective against many diseases, such as gonorrhea, syphilis, and meningitis. Fleming was knighted in 1944 and won the Nobel Prize in physiology for his extraordinary achievements and contribution to the advancement of medical sciences.

A microbiologist by the name of Selman Waksman discovered streptomycin in 1943. Streptomycin was the first antibiotic that was effective against tuberculosis as well as many other bacterial infections.

The 1930s saw the introduction of sulfonamides that were applied directly to wounds; topical penicillin appeared in 1943. Corticosteroids and steroid creams were used to treat inflammatory skin conditions until the inhibitory effect of cortisone on wound healing was discovered in 1964 by Sandberg.

Other antiseptic solutions that were in use in the 1940's included ethyl alcohol, colloidal silver, acetic acid, boric acid, genetian violet, hexachlorophene, and thimerosol. In vitro research after the war suggested that these agents were cytotoxic to human cells, and clinicians therefore became reluctant to use them.

For the next fifty-plus years, antibiotics cured many illnesses and saved countless lives. Because of their success in fighting infections, however, they have been overprescribed and misused. The result of this misuse has created new superbugs known as resistant bacteria.

The staph aureas bacterium was first discovered in the 1880s. It not only causes painful skin lesions and impetigo but can progress to bacterial pneumonia and septicemia, both of which can be fatal. As staph aureas developed resistance to penicillin in the 1940s and 1950s, a new drug called methicillin was found to treat it. The magic soon wore off as British scientists identified the first strains of staph aureas that were immune to methicillin in 1961, thus heralding in the new era of methicillin-resistant staph aureas (MRSA).

Other penicillin-like antibiotics, called beta-lactams, were used. As the staph aureas bacteria continue to evolve, it is showing resistance to these other antibiotics as well. In 2002, U.S. physicians documented the first case of staph aureas that is immune to vancomycin, currently the last resort in the fight against one of the most common sepsis-causing agents of all time.

Because the history of sepsis dates far back into ancient times, it is impossible to estimate how many lives have been taken by these nearly invisible pathogens. Currently, sepsis-causing bacterium cost more than $20 billion annually to the US healthcare system and adds more than 8 million days in the hospital. (Hughes, 2011) Even though we have progressive standards of living in the US and many other countries, worldwide 15,000,000 children die every year from preventable infectious diseases. Simple medical treatments, immunization, and basic sanitation could prevent a majority of these deaths. (Hulbert, 1999)

Theories on sepsis and wound-care management have been studied and written about for thousands of years. Evidence suggests that sepsis dates back further than even our written records indicate. Numerous methods of treatment have been discovered, along with countless different herbs and treatments that have been experimented with as we continue to battle the many invisible pathogens.

We nurses are at the bedside 24 hours per day. We perform physical assessments, take vital signs, and have almost continuous hands-on communication with our patients. We nurses will be the first to notice the first signs of sepsis and to alert the physicians. We must be able to recognize the early signs of sepsis in order to begin treatment. Becoming aware of the history of this elusive enemy and realizing the insidious nature of disease-causing pathogens is the first step in our fight against sepsis.

References

1. Hughes, James M. (2011). Preserving the Lifesaving Power of Antimicrobial Agents. *JAMA* 305 (10), 1027-1028. Retrieved from http://jama.jamanetwork.com/article.aspx?volume=305&issue=10&page=1027 .

2. Hulbert, R. E. (1999). *Microbiology 101/102.* Retrieved from http://www.slic2.wsu.edu:82/hurlbert/ micro101/pages/chap1.html

3. Miller, Jason T., Rahimi, Scott Y., and Lee, Mark. (2005) History of Infection Control and Its Contributions to the Development and Success of Brain Tumor Operations. *American Association of Neurological Surgeons* 2005, 18 (4) 1-5. Retrieved from http://www.medscape.com/ viewarticle/503947

4. Mouës, Chantal M., Heule, Freerk, Legerstee, Ron, and Hovius, Steven. (2009). Five Millennia of Wound

Care Products—What Is New? A Literature Review. *Ostomy Wound Management* 55 (3), 16-32. Retrieved from http://www.o-wm.com/content/five-millennia-wound-care-products-%E2%80%94-what-new-a-literature-review

CHAPTER 3

Common Organisms

SEPSIS CAN BE CAUSED BY many different organisms such as bacteria, fungi, viruses, or parasites. Blood is normally sterile, and when an organism invades, the infection is called bacteremia, fungemia, viremia, or parasitemia, depending on the invading organism. An organism can be either widespread, when it is in the blood, or limited to a particular region, as in a tooth abscess. Some bacteria, such as staphylococcus, live on the skin. They are harmless unless a break in the skin allows them to enter the bloodstream, where they can cause the potentially fatal toxic shock syndrome. E. coli is another bacterium that is perfectly harmless in the gastrointestinal tract but that can be fatal if it gets into the bloodstream.

The following list includes common infections that can lead to sepsis, especially in people with poorly functioning immune systems such that a local infection can overwhelm the body and invade the bloodstream.

- Cellulitis (skin infection) of face, ear, arm, hand, leg, foot, abdomen, or breast

- Cholecystitis (gallbladder inflammation)
- Colitis (inflammation of the inner lining of the colon)
- Endocarditis (inflammation of the inner lining of the heart)
- Gangrene (death of body tissue from bacterial infection or lack of blood flow)
- Meningitis (inflammation of brain and/or spinal cord)
- Osteomyelitis (infection of the bone)
- Perforated bowel (a hole in the wall of the stomach that leaks contents into the abdomen)
- Peritonitis (inflammation of the tissue that lines the interior of the abdomen)
- Pneumonia (lung infection)
- Pyelonephritis (kidney infection)
- Urinary tract infection
- Septic arthritis (disease-causing organisms spread to a joint)

Bacteria are the most abundant of all organisms. They are single-celled microorganisms that live either as independent life forms or as parasites (living off other life forms). Being single-celled means that they have no nucleus or any other membrane-bound organelles. Bacteria are considered to be primitive organisms, as they share many features of other living organisms, such as being composed of cells; needing to get energy from the environment to exist, grow, and reproduce; transmitting genetic information via DNA; and exhibiting sexual reproduction (only some do this).

Bacteria are found everywhere on earth: in the air and soil, in hot and cold temperatures, and from the depths of the oceans to the tops of the tallest mountains. They congregate where they have what they need to survive, such as

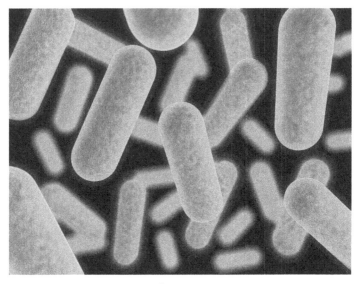

Bacteria.

food, moisture, and the right temperature in which to flourish and grow.

Ferdinand Cohn was a German botanist (1828–1898) who came up with the name bacteria. He based it on the Greek work *bakterion*, which means a small rod or staff. In 1853, Cohn categorized bacteria according to their shape: bacteria (short rods), bacilli (longer rods), and spirella (spiral formations). Other ways to categorize bacteria are based on their cell-wall characteristics and their patterns of growth, as in the chains formed by streptococci.

Cell-wall characteristics are identified by using the gram stain. A Danish bacteriologist named Christian Gram discovered that when bacteria are placed on a slide, heated, and dipped in a blue dye, the gram-positive bacteria retain the blue color. The colorless gram-negative bacteria do not retain the blue dye. The slide is then counterstained with a red dye, which makes the gram-negative bacteria appear red. The cell walls of gram-positive and gram-negative bacteria are similar, but the gram-positive cell wall is thicker and more sensitive to dyes and antibiotics, and the gram-negative cell wall is sandwiched between an inner cell membrane and an outer lipid-containing cell membrane.

The human body provides a perfect environment for billions of microorganisms to call home. They live on our skin, in our mouths and noses, and in our gastrointestinal (GI) tracts. Not all bacteria that coexist with us are harmful, however. For example, lactobacillus acidophilus lives in the intestines of humans. It destroys disease-causing organisms while helping our bodies digest food. More than 400 other beneficial bacteria live in the human GI tract. They help keep us healthy by digesting foods and helping to eliminate wastes.

The healthy probiotic bacteria in the human body decrease with age, and a number of unhealthy lifestyle habits decrease them further. Such habits include excessive alcohol consumption, stress, and poor diet.

Some bacteria are used in combination with other yeasts and molds to help in the fermentation process of some foods such as cheese, yogurt, wine, vinegar, sauerkraut, and pickles. These bacteria do more than aid in fermentation; they are high in enzymes, improve digestion and absorption of nutrients, and enhance the flavors of foods.

Gram-negative bacteria used to be the main cause for sepsis, but gram-positive bacteria have now taken the lead. In an online article on sepsis by Jessica Ryon, these are listed as the most common causative organisms:

- Gram-positive bacteria 52.9%
- Gram-negative bacteria 41.6%
- Fungi 4.1%
- Anaerobic organisms 1.4% (Ryon, n.d.)

Gram-negative bacteria are normal residents of the GI system, and they cause disease only when they invade other areas. Of the total gram-negative sepsis-causing agents, E. coli is responsible in 40% of cases; Klebsiella-Enterobacteriaceae-Serratia in 20%; pseudomonas aeruginosa in 20%; Bacteriodes in 10%; and Proteus also in 10%. (Wahl, n.d.)

Common Community-Acquired Organisms

- Escherichia coli
- Staphylococcus aureus
- Streptococcus pneumonia

Common Hospital-Acquired Organisms

- Gram-negative aerobic bacilli
- Coagulase-negative staphylococcus
- Staphylococcus aureus
- Enterococci
- Candida

Bacteria That Commonly Cause Sepsis

- Acinetobacter species
- Clostridium difficile
- Escherichia coli
- Enterobacter species
- Enterococcus species
- Haemophilus influenza
- Klebsiella species
- Listeria monocytogenes
- Neisseria meningitis
- Pseudomonas aeruginosa

- Serratia species
- Staphylococcus species
- Streptococcus species

Fungi

Molds, mildew, and yeast are forms of fungi, a type of parasitic plant. There are approximately 100,000 different types of fungi, with 50 of them able to cause disease in humans. Fungal infections occur in warm, moist, dark areas where there is little to no air flow and on skin that is irritated, constantly moist, or weakened in some way. The fungi are able to multiply and invade areas such as the skin, GI tract, genitals, lungs, liver, or any other areas on the body.

Dermatophytes are a group of fungi that rarely penetrate below the skin. They cause redness, itching, scaling, peeling, blistering, and brittle hair and nails.

Common Types of Fungal Infections (Dermatophytes)

- Tinea Pedis—Athlete's Foot. Found between the toes and/or on the bottom of the foot.
- Tinea Capitis—Ringworm on the scalp. Found on the scalp and/or hair. Occurs mostly in children.
- Tinea Barbae—Barber's Itch. Found on the bearded part of the face.
- Tinea Corporis—Ringworm. Found anywhere on the body.
- Tinea Cruris—Jock Itch. Found from the groin area to the inner thigh.
- Tinea unguium—Onychomycosis – fungal nails. Affects toenails and fingernails.

Malassezia furfur, though not a dermatophyte, is yeast that causes Tinea versicolor, which are multicolored lesions or patches on the skin that occur commonly in young adults.

Another fungal infection of the skin that is not caused by a dermatophyte is sporothrix schenckii. This infection occurs when thorny plants that harbor the fungus, such as pine needles or sphagnum moss, scratch the skin or subcutaneous tissue.

Candida is a flora found in the mouth. It is also one of the most common yeast infections. An overgrowth of candida albicans is called candidiasis. It causes redness and white patches in the mouth known as thrush. In babies, candida is the cause of diaper rash, and in women, it can occur as a vaginal infection. It can often indicate an underlying disease process such as diabetes mellitus, malignant tumor, or chronic infection.

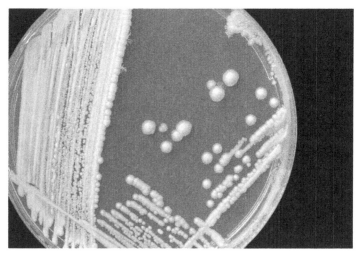

Fungal colony of candida albicans.

According to an article in Lab Tests Online, The Centers for Disease Control (CDC) states that "almost 75% of women will have at least one yeast infection in their lifetime", and that candidiasis as the fourth most common cause of hospital-acquired septicemia in the United States. (2011)

The use of antibiotics can trigger or enhance a yeast infection, as antibiotics interrupt the balance of normal flora in the body. If not treated, thrush in the mouth can travel down the esophagus and into the GI tract, then into the bloodstream, where it has a 70% fatality rate. The bottom line is that a yeast infection must be spotted and treated quickly.

Following is a list of common deep or systemic fungal infections and where they are commonly found.

- Aspergillosis—house dust, soil, and plants
- Blastomycosis—moist organic-rich soil of southeastern and south central United States
- Coccidiomycosis—arid soil of southwest United States, Mexico, and South America (an infection of the lungs that produces excessive sputum and nodules)
- Cryptococcosis—soil associated with bird droppings (may infect anyone, but people with HIV/AIDS are at highest risk)
- Histoplasmosis—eastern and central United States (affects primarily the lungs)
- Candidiasis—worldwide (occurs in moist mucous membranes)
- Pneumocystis (formerly known as Pneumocystis carinii)—worldwide (occurs most in immune-compromised people, such as those with HIV/AIDS)

In addition to bacteria and fungi, viruses also cause many diseases. Viruses are tiny particles that are 1000 times smaller than bacteria and much smaller than human cells. In fact, viruses are so small; they can be seen only with electron microscopes. Viruses are basically small capsules shaped like rods, spheres, or tadpoles that contain only genetic material. They are not able to eat, grow, or reproduce on their own like normal human cells or bacteria. Instead, they lie around their environment, waiting for a host cell to invade and grow in, which results in the death of the host cell.

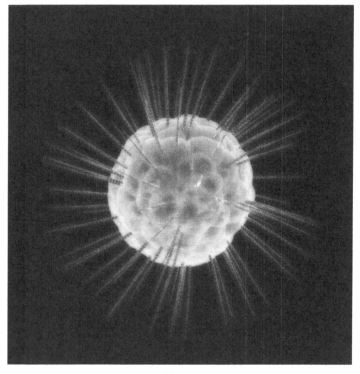

Virus.

Some Common Viruses

- AIDS
- Influenza
- Measles
- Smallpox
- Common cold
- Ebola hemorrhagic fever
- Genital herpes

Some viruses, such as HIV and herpes, mix their own genetic instructions right into the host cell's genetic instructions. In this way, when the host cell reproduces, the virus's genetic code is copied instead. The virus can basically sleep this way for years while the host has many rounds of reproductive cycles, until some event or environmental factor wakes the virus up. This is known as the lysogenic cycle. This is why some people who are infected with the HIV virus can live for years and not know they are sick; in the meantime, they can infect anyone with whom they may have intimate.

How Viruses Attack

1. A person who is already infected sneezes or coughs near you.
2. The virus particle attaches to the lining of your sinuses when you breathe it in.
3. The virus rapidly grows and reproduces after it attacks the cells lining your sinuses.
4. The host cells break, allowing the virus to enter your bloodstream and lungs.
5. The virus travels down your throat, making the throat sore, and the loss of the lining in the sinuses causes a runny nose.

6. The virus attacks different muscles, making them sore.
7. Chemicals called pyrogens are produced and increase your body temperature.

Because viruses invade host cells, they are protected from medicines such as antibiotics. Only a few antiviral medicines are available at this time.

Sepsis can occur in any part of the body. The most common regions are listed below.

- The lungs—Sepsis in the lungs is usually associated with pneumonia from a hospital-acquired infection.
- The abdomen—Sepsis can begin in many possible ways in the abdomen, such as gallbladder infections, appendicitis, or peritonitis when the outer surfaces of the abdominal organs are involved.
- Kidney, bladder, or urinary tract—Diabetics and those with catheters are at highest risk for urinary tract infections.
- The skin—Wounds, skin breakdown or inflammation, and IV sites are the most Common sources of sepsis in the skin.
- Bones—Bones, bone marrow, and sinuses are sites of infections.
- Central nervous system—Sepsis can begin with inflammation and/or infection of the brain or spinal cord, as in meningitis or encephalitis.

In about 20% of cases, the source of sepsis is never discovered.

Parasites are the final common type of organism that can cause sepsis. Parasites are similar to viruses in that they require a host to get their nourishment and protection. They are found worldwide in contaminated food, water, fruits, vegetables, meats, and soil. They are a common source of food and waterborne illnesses.

Parasites are easily transmitted by having the feces of an infected person or animal touch the mouth, such as when a pet licks your face or you eat contaminated food. These transmissions can occur from human to human, from human to animal, or from animal to human. Because humans can be host to more than 100 types of parasites, the symptoms of a parasitic infection are varied and wide-spread:

- Anemia—As the parasites suck out vital nutrients, they can cause iron deficiency.
- Allergies—Increased foreign proteins can cause inflammation and allergic reactions to certain foods.
- Digestive disturbances—Gas and bloating can be caused by worms that live in the upper intestines.
- Growths—Tumors and cysts can be formed from parasites that clump together.
- Fatigue—Chronic fatigue and flu-like symptoms can include apathy and depression.
- Restlessness and nervous energy—These can be caused by parasitic waste that irritates the central nervous system. Verminous waste can also cause unclear thinking, dizziness, high or low blood sugar, and poor digestion.

The size of a parasite can vary from large, like a worm, and visible to the naked eye to very small, like single-celled organisms called protozoa, and more difficult to see. Not only is parasites' size variable; so are their lifestyles. Some live on one permanent host, whereas others can experience different human and/or animal hosts as they pass through a series of developmental phases.

Types of Parasites

Roundworms

Roundworms include hookworms, whipworms, pinworms, trichinosis, dog heartworms, Toxocara Canis, and the common roundworm. An estimated 25% of people worldwide are infected with roundworms. Roundworm infection is caused by eating the worm eggs that are on fruits and vegetables. Symptoms include blood sugar imbalances, anemia, intestinal gas, fatigue, anemia, and weight gain around the full moon.

Tapeworms

Tapeworms include pork tapeworm, dwarf tapeworm, broad fish tapeworm, beef tapeworm, and rat tapeworm.

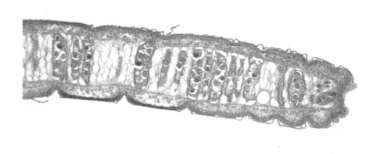

Tapeworm.

Tapeworms are found worldwide. They can grow to be very large, and there are many different species. Tapeworms can be contracted by eating tapeworm eggs or from intermediate hosts such as beef, pork, or fish. They live in the intestines and absorb vital nutrients such as vitamin B-12 and folic acid. Symptoms of tapeworm infection include jaundice, intestinal gas, thyroid imbalances, bloating, and fluid buildup during the full moon.

Flukes

Flukes include metagonemus, opisthorchis, Schistosoma, Fasciola, heterophyes, Paragonimus, and dicrocoelium.

Flukes are smaller parasites and attach themselves to different organs. Flukes can be contracted by eating raw or undercooked fish, eating infected vegetables, or wading through or drinking infected water. Symptoms of fluke infection include inflammation and damage to organs such as the lungs, liver, bladder, blood vessels, heart, or brain.

Single-Celled Parasites

Single-celled parasites include protozoa, Toxoplasma, amoeba, Giardia, neospora, Trichomonas, and Cryptosporidium. They are microscopic in size and harm more people than any other parasitic disease, as they are found everywhere in our environment. Exposure is common; however, healthy immune systems can fight them easily. Symptoms are like those associated with asthma, psoriasis, arthritis, degenerative muscle diseases, multiple sclerosis, ovarian cysts, and lymphomas.

Parasites are very smart. They know that they need hosts to survive, and once inside humans, they secretly feed off the energy, nourishment, and cells of the body.

People can live for years with parasitic infections and never know that they are harboring a parallel life. That's the secret to parasites' success: They make us only a little sick so we think it's just a normal process of aging that is causing us to feel bad. The majority of people don't even know they have an infection, and most of them may never even seek treatment.

References

1. Fungal Infections. (n.d.). Lab Tests Online. from http://www.labtestsonline.org/understanding/conditions/fungal-2.html
2. Ryon, Jessica. (n.d.). *Sepsis*. Retrieved from http://www.austincc.edu/microbio/2704j/sepsis.htm
3. Wahl, Sharon. (n.d.). *Septic Shock: How to Detect It Early*. Retrieved from http://www2.hawaii.edu/~johnb/micro/m130/readings/SepticShock.htm

CHAPTER 4

Risk Factors for Sepsis

EVEN THOUGH SEPSIS CAN OCCUR in anyone who already has an infection, some factors increase the risk of acquiring sepsis:

1. Age: Includes infants and people over the age of 60.
2. Compromised immune system: Includes people who are battling other disease processes such as cancer or AIDS, people who are taking anti-rejection drugs from receiving an organ transplant, and people with kidney or liver failure.
3. Hospitalization: Includes people who are already in the hospital.
4. Invasive medical equipment: Includes people with equipment such as indwelling urinary catheters, IV access (especially central line or dialysis catheters), or endotracheal tubes for life support.
5. Disease: Includes people with diabetes.

6. Steroid use: Includes people taking high doses of steroids.
7. Insurance status: A newly released study by Ohio State University Medical Center states that patients who are insured by Medicare or Medicaid are at a higher risk of being hospitalized with sepsis than those with private insurance. (Obrien et al., 2011)
8. Race: Black people have a higher risk of contracting sepsis than do Hispanics or whites. Other factors mentioned in this article include male gender, low income zip codes, and urban residence (Gever, 2008).
9. Surgery history. Includes people who've recently needed emergency surgery.
10. Neutropenia: People with neutropenia have a decrease in a type of white blood cell that is the first to fight infection.

Sepsis can be a very costly complication to a hospital visit. Often, when a person is undergoing surgery or other disease-fighting procedures, his or her immune system becomes weakened and the person is at a much higher risk of acquiring sepsis. Knowing which persons are at higher risk can help healthcare providers be extra cautious and vigilant in observing for signs of infection. Recovery improves dramatically when sepsis is identified and treated quickly. According to a prospective observational study in England, "Non-compliance with the six hour sepsis bundle was associated with a more than twofold increase in hospital mortality." (Gao, Melody, Daniels, Giles, & Fox, 2005)

References

1. Gao, Fang., Melody, Teresa., Daniels, Darren F., Giles, Simon., & Fox, Samantha (2005). The impact of compliance with 6-hour and 24-hour sepsis bundles on hospital mortality in patients with severe sepsis: a prospective observational study. *Critical Care*, 9, R764-R770. Retrieved from http://www.biomedcentral.com/content/pdf/cc3909. pdf

2. Gever, John (2008, February 1). Higher Sepsis Rate Among Blacks Supersedes Risk Factors. *Medpage Today*. Retrieved from http://www.medpagetoday. com/InfectiousDisease/GeneralInfectiousDisease/ 8180

3. O'Brien, James M., Lu, Bo, Naeem, A. Ali, Levine, Deborah A., Aberegg, Scott K., & Lemeshow, Stanley (2011). Insurance type and sepsis-associated mortality among US adults: A retrospective cohort study. *Critical Care* 15, 3

CHAPTER 5

Preventing Sepsis

AS WE'VE SEEN, MANY PATHOGENS can cause sepsis. Bacteria, fungi, viruses, and parasites live and grow in the environment all around us. Everywhere we turn, everything we eat and do, puts us at risk of contracting an infection. Undercooked meat, unwashed fruits and vegetables, contaminated water, and even the normal flora on our skin can invade us and turn deadly.

Our immune systems are constantly under attack from these unseen organisms. The very best thing we as individuals can do to keep healthy is to help our immune systems in that fight. Some things, such as being treated with chemotherapy or having autoimmune diseases, can't be helped, but the general public can take several actions to protect themselves.

- Eat healthily. Limit simple sugars, saturated fats, and empty-calorie foods.
- Stay active. Studies prove that people who are more active and physically fit are the least likely to

suffer from colds in winter months. (Lavelle, 2010).
- Get plenty of rest.
- Don't smoke.
- Avoid excessive alcohol.
- Maintain a healthy blood pressure and body weight.
- Cook meats thoroughly, to a minimum internal temperature of 145 degrees.
- Drink water only from treated municipal water supplies, when hiking or camping. Avoid drinking water directly from lakes, ponds, or other non-treated sources. If you travel out of the country, be sure to boil the water at least one minute before drinking to kill any flora that your body is not accustomed to.
- Drink only pasteurized milk, juice, and ciders.
- Wash, peel, and/or cook raw fruits and vegetables.
- (Women only) Change tampons at least every 3–4 hours and use the least absorbent ones required to prevent toxic shock syndrome.
- Get vaccinated. Even though many previously well-known diseases are now rare because of our vigilant vaccination practices, they would soon return if we stopped giving routine vaccines ("Why Immunize", 2012).

There are many different vaccination schedules for people of different ages, including 0–6 years of age, 7–18 years of age, and 19 years and older. A catch-up schedule exists for those aged 4 months to 18 years who have started vaccinations late or are more than one month behind. (Recommended Immunization Schedules for Persons Aged 0 Through 18 Years – United States, 2012).

Childhood Vaccines

1. Measles
2. Tetanus (Lockjaw)
3. Rubella (German measles)
4. Diphtheria
5. Hepatitis A
6. Hepatitis B
7. Pertussis (Whooping cough)
8. Pneumococcal disease (Causes bacterial meningitis and blood infections)
9. Human papillomavirus
10. Rotovirus
11. Polio
12. Haemophilus influenza type B (Hib; a major cause of bacterial meningitis)
13. Meningococcal disease
14. Mumps
15. Varicella

Adult Vaccines (for those aged 19 and above)

1. Diphtheria
2. Herpes zoster (Shingles)
3. Influenza (Flu)
4. Pneumococcus
5. Tetanus (Lockjaw)
6. Pertussis (Whooping cough)
7. Varicella
8. Human papillomavirus
9. Zoster
10. Measles, mumps, and rubella (MMR)
11. Hepatitis A
12. Hepatitis B

By keeping yourself healthy, you may be able to combat an infection and thereby stop the spread of possible epidemic diseases.

Nursing Interventions to Prevent Sepsis

1. Wash your hands thoroughly before and after patient contact. Several studies have found that there is just as much risk of gloves becoming contaminated from the environment as there is in touching an infected patient. In other words, the germs are in the room and on the surfaces of the environment, it doesn't matter if you touch the patient or not – you could still have the germs on your hands. Furthermore, hand washing compliance is still only around 50%, even in intensive care areas. (The Healthcare Environment- Hand washing is not enough, 2012).

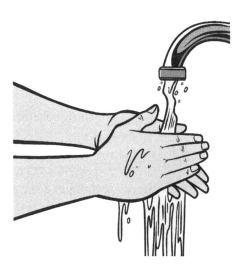

Washing your hands before treating patients is extremely important.

2. Use personal protective equipment such as goggles, gowns, and gloves as needed. Wear goggles to protect your eyes from body fluids or other debris, gowns to protect your clothes from getting soiled, and gloves for every patient contact.

3. Follow hospital policy with IV and central venous catheter site care.

    • Most hospitals advise the use of chlorhexidine skin preparation for IV site care. This includes not only for peripheral IV insertions but also when assisting with central venous catheters (CVC) and their routine site care. Manufacturers' suggestions are to allow the chlorhexidine to dry for two minutes before handling the site. (Donnelly, Foster, & Bannon, 2007)

    • Monitor IV sites daily for redness or drainage. Change peripheral IVs per hospital policy and notify the doctor at once if signs of infection appear. Change IV dressings when they become loose or soiled, and clean the area well per hospital policy. Clean the hub of the IV tubing well with alcohol before it is accessed each time, whether to give a medication or to draw blood.

4. Provide proper indwelling urethral catheter care.

    • Wash hands before and after catheter insertion.

    • Use strict sterile technique during insertion.

    • Maintain an unobstructed urine flow, and never place Foley bag higher than the level of the patient. Leave the bag hanging on the bedside for all road trips and transfers.

- Maintain a closed drainage system. Many catheters now have an extra port to flush or obtain a urine sample from. Again, clean the hub well with alcohol and allow it to dry before you access it.
- Be sure to discontinue the indwelling catheter as soon as it is no longer needed. Catheter-associated urinary tract infections (CAUTIs) account for 32% of the 2 million healthcare-associated infections every year, and 80% of those are due to indwelling urethral catheters. The annual cost is estimated to be $565 million in the United States alone. (Safety Leaders, n.d.)

5. Strive to prevent ventilator-associated pneumonia. The second most common nosocomial infection in the United States is pneumonia, and patients who receive mechanical ventilation for more than 48 hours can acquire what is called ventilator-assisted pneumonia (VAP). VAP increases length of stay in ICU by as much as 5–7 days, adds an additional $40,000 per hospital admission, and costs an estimated $1.2 billion per year. (Augustyn, 2007)
   - Wash hands thoroughly before putting on gloves and making contact with patient.
   - Elevate head of bed to 30–45 degrees to prevent aspiration.
   - Minimize sedation to help facilitate faster weaning.
   - Ensure that pharmacological agents are used to enhance gastric motility and prevent gastric distention.
   - Provide frequent oral care, including suctioning secretions from the back of throat and

using oral decontamination such as chlorhexidine.

- Avoid saline lavage.
- Turn patients at least every 2 hours to promote tracheal drainage.
- Maintain endotracheal cuff pressure of 20cm H2O.
- Ensure that a stress ulcer prophylaxis is in use.
- Monitor the residual volumes on gastric tubes to prevent gastric distention.

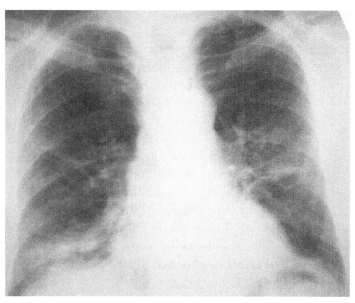

Septic pneumonia.

Organisms exist in the world all around us. They are hungry to attack and to invade us and live off our life energy. Practice healthy lifestyle habits to minimize the severity of any illness, and follow universal precautions to decrease the risk of spreading disease.

References

1. Augustyn, Beth. (2007). Ventilator-Associated Pneumonia: Risk Factors and Prevention. *Critical Care Nurse*. 27, (4) 32-36. Retrieved from http://www.scribd.com/doc/46254891/VAP-Risk-Factors-and-Prevention

3. Centers for Disease Control and Prevention. (2012). Recommended Immunization Schedules for Persons Aged 0 Through 18 Years – United States, 2012. Retrieved from http://www.cdc.gov/vaccines/schedules/downloads/child/mmwr-child-schedule.pdf

4. Centers for Disease Control and Prevention. (2012). The healthcare Environment – Hand Washing is Not Enough. Retrieved from http://bio-intervention.com/problem/hand-washing.html

5. Centers for Disease Control and Prevention. (2012). Why Immunize? Retrieved from http://www.cdc.gov/vaccines/vac-gen/why.htm

5. Donnelly, Stephanie Francis., Foster, Shannon Marie., & Bannon, Michael P. (2007). 5 Steps to prevent CVC-related infections. *Contemporary Surgery*, 63, (12), 600-604. Retrieved from http://www.contemporarysurgery.com/pdf/6312/6312CS_Review.pdf

6. Lavelle, Peter. (2010, November 2). Study proves exercise boosts immune system. *ABC Science*. Retrieved from http://www.abc.net.au/science/articles/2010/11/02/ 3054621.htm

6. Safety Leaders, (n.d.). *Quickstart for SP #25: Catheter-Associated Urinary Tract Infection Prevention*. Retrieved from http://www.safetyleaders.org/pages/QuickStart.jsp?step=0&spnum=25

CHAPTER 6

The Sepsis Cascade and Multiple-Organ Dysfunction Syndrome (MODS)

Glossary of Terms

Activated Protein C—Inhibits the production of pro-inflammatory cytokines

Acute Tubular Necrosis—A kidney injury caused by toxic medications, antifungal agents, radiology dye, or lack of oxygen. It can lead to kidney failure.

Apoptosis—Programmed cell death; a dominant process that stops inflammation after an infection has subsided

Bacteremia—A situation in which bacteria is in the blood (not the same as sepsis).

Baroreceptors—Pressure-sensitive nerve endings found in the walls in the atria of the heart, the aortic arch, and the carotid sinuses. Baroreceptors are stimulated by changes in blood pressure and allow for physiologic adjustments to help maintain homeostasis.

Compensatory anti-inflammatory reaction (CARS)—A systematic deactivation of the immune system in response to a severe infection, that tries to restore homeostasis from an inflammatory state.

Complement system—A protein cascade that helps clear pathogens from an organism.

Cytokines—Polypeptide regulators that carry signals for cellular communication. Cytokines are often secreted in response to invading pathogens to activate other immune system fighter cells.

Fibrinolysis—The breakdown of fibrin clots.

Interferon—A protein that interferes with viruses.

Interleukins—A group of naturally occurring proteins that regulate cell growth, motility, and differentiation, as well as mediate communication between cells. Interleukins play a major role in stimulating the immune responses, such as with inflammation.

Microvascular permeability—A condition that allows leaking of capillary walls.

Multiple organ dysfunction syndrome (MODS)—Altered organ function in a critically ill patient who can't maintain homeostasis.

Pattern-recognition receptors—Cells that recognize specific structures of microorganisms and initiate the innate immune system response.

Phagocytes—White blood cells, leukocytes, and monocytes that can engulf and digest foreign particles.

Platelet activating factor (PAF)—A lipid mediator that causes platelet aggregation, inflammation, and other allergic responses.

Polymorphonuclear leukocytes (PMNs)—A form of white blood cells. PMNs express adhesion molecules that migrate to the site of cellular injury to cause aggregation and margination to the vascular endothelium.

Systemic inflammatory response syndrome (SIRS)—A severe systemic response to an injury or insult such as trauma, infection, or burn that is characterized by a group of two or more expected symptoms (elevated heart rate, abnormally high or low temperature, high respiratory rate or low level of carbon dioxide in blood, and high or low white blood cell count with more than 10% neutrophils).

Thromboxane—A substance made by platelets that causes blood clotting and blood vessels to constrict.

Tumor necrosis factor (TNF)—Produced by macrophages; kills tumor cells and promotes creation of new blood cells.

The immune system is a group of cells and organs that work together to fight off invading organisms. The first line of defense is the skin. It forms a layer of protection that prevents organisms from entering. It also secretes antibacterial substances that destroys bacteria and molds that land on the body. Tears, mucous, and saliva are the second line of defense preventing organisms from entering the body. Lysozyme is an enzyme in tears and mucous that breaks down the cell walls of many bacteria (discovered in 1921 by Alexander Fleming, who was mentioned in Chapter 1). Many forms of bacteria and viruses are swept away by these fluids.

If an organism does gain entry into the body, the immune system is responsible for eradicating that organism. The following components work together to eradicate invading organisms and to return the body to homeostasis (the normal state, when the body is healthy and there is balance between coagulation and fibrinolysis):

- Bone marrow—produces red and white blood cells.

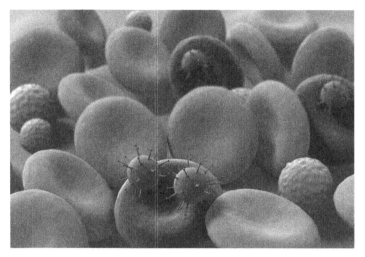

Red and white blood cells with virus.

- Spleen—filters foreign matter and old red blood cells from the blood.
- White blood cells—consists of many different types that each have their own function, such as neutrophils, eosinophils, basophils, monocytes, and lymphocytes. Neutrophils are the most abundant form and they kill bacteria in the body by process known as phagocytosis. Eosinophils release toxins that kill parasites. Basophils assist with the inflammatory response. Monocytes are the largest type of white blood cell and they help clean the foreign particles after an inflammatory response. The final type of white blood cell is called a lymphocyte, and these are involved in the last stage of the immune system that allows long term resistance to a repeated infection.

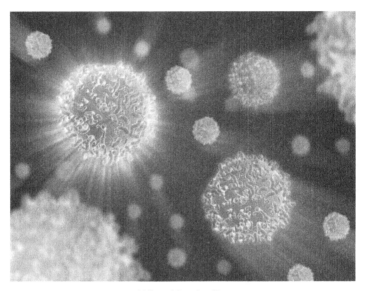

White blood cells.

- Thymus—produces T-cells (one of the white blood cells).
- Lymph—clear, watery fluid that detects and removes waste products.
- Lymph nodes—are filters that trap debris such as bacteria, viruses, cancer cells and other dead tissue to be eliminated from the body.
- Antibodies—substances produced by white blood cells. Antibodies include proteins called immunoglobulins and gamma globulins, proteins that bind to invading toxins (antigens) and disable them.
- Hormones—cytokines that are very potent chemical messengers secreted by different cells and that can perform a variety of functions depending on their origin.

- Complement system—a series of proteins that are manufactured by the liver, float freely through the blood, and work with antibodies to lyse (burst) cells to be removed by phagocytes.

Organisms can gain entry into the body in many ways: through a break in the skin, through the lungs, or in what is eaten and drunk. Organisms can even travel through the genitourinary tract after sex or after contact with a contaminated surface. As the organism spreads and gains entry into the bloodstream, it triggers a systemic inflammatory response known as sepsis, which includes coagulopathy, hypotension, inadequate tissue perfusion, organ failure, and death.

At the local site of injury, there will be inflammation, edema, and increased micro vascular permeability. Phagocytes secrete cytokines such as TNF and interleukins that will regulate the local inflammatory process. Cytokine levels are further increased by the self-stimulating TNF. This results in the release of other inflammatory mediators such as platelet-activating factor (PAF), interferon, eicosanoids, and interleukins 1,2,6,8, and 10. As more polymorphonuclear leukocytes are recruited, the invading organism and resulting debris are cleared away and tissue repair begins. (Neviere, 2011) Sepsis occurs when polymorphonuclear leukocyte release exceeds the boundaries of the local environment, which results in a more generalized immune-system response.

These pro-inflammatory mediators facilitate inflammation, promote coagulation, inhibit fibrinolysis, and activate other cells that initiate the sepsis cascade that results in endothelial damage. Once this inflammatory response has been initiated, it causes vasodilation and microvascular permeability, which in turn causes blood clots to form on the vessel walls.

In an effort to assist with tissue repair and healing, a release of anti-inflammatory elements that try to maintain homeostasis occurs simultaneously with the inflammatory cascade of SIRS. Systemic inflammatory response syndrome (SIRS) occurs from the excessive pro-inflammatory response, whereas compensatory anti-inflammatory reaction syndrome (CARS) is the result of inappropriate immunosuppression. Sometimes, these opposing elements of SIRS and CARS balance each other to result in homeostasis; however, often, by interfering with each other's attempts, they create a state of destructive immunologic dissonance.

Normally, fibrinolysis will break down blood clots and assist in healing the wound, but in a sepsis condition, fibrinolysis does not occur. Microscopic blood clots then occlude the blood flow to extremities and vital organs, causing tissue hypoxia and organ death.

Pro-inflammatory Mediators

Free radical generation
HMGB1 protein
H2S
IFN-
IL-1 , IL-2,IL-6, IL-8, IL-15
Neutrophil elastase
NO
Phospholipase A2
PAF
Plasminogen activator inhibitor-1
Prostacyclin
Prostaglandins
Protein kinase
Soluble adhesion molecules
Thromboxane

TNF-
Tyrosine kinase
Vasoactive neuropeptides

Anti-inflammatory Mediators

Epinephrine
IL-1Ra
IL-4
IL-10
IL-13
Leukotriene B4-receptor antagonist
LPS binding protein
Soluble recombinant CD-14
Soluble TNF-α receptors
Transforming growth factor-β
Type II IL-1 receptor

Blood pressure drops in response to the decreased circulation. Baroreceptors in the aorta and in the carotid arteries recognize the lowering blood pressure and activate the sympathetic nervous system. Potent vasoconstrictors such as epinephrine and norepinephrine are released to increase circulation and provide adequate blood flow to the vital organs—the heart and brain. At the same time, blood is shunted away from the non-vital organs (including the kidneys, lungs, skin, and GI tract). When the kidneys recognize the decreased blood flow, they initiate the renin-angiotensin-aldosterone system that results in worsening cardiac output and lowers circulating volume, and the blood pressure drops further. This process creates an irreversible condition that leads to multiple-organ dysfunction syndrome (MODS) and death.

According to the American College of Chest Physicians/Society of Critical Care Medicine consensus panel, sepsis has different levels of severity beginning with systemic inflammatory response syndrome (SIRS), sepsis, severe sepsis, septic shock, or multiple organ dysfunction syndrome, each with its own requirements and definitions. (Picard, O'Donoghue, Young-Kershaw, & Russell, 2006)

Systemic Inflammatory Response Syndrome (SIRS)

SIRS is a widespread inflammatory response to a variety of injuries such as pancreatitis, trauma, and burns. It is manifested by two or more of the following conditions:

- Temperature >38°C or <36°C
- Heart rate >90 bpm
- Respiratory rate >20/min or PaCO2<32 mm Hg
- White blood cell count >12 x 109/L or <4 x109/L, or with >10% immature (band) forms

Sepsis: There is definite evidence of infection, along with the clinical signs of SIRS

Severe Sepsis: Sepsis with hypo-perfusion, hypotension, or organ dysfunction. Clinical signs may include oliguria, altered mental status changes, and increased lactic acidosis.

Septic Shock: Along with signs of severe sepsis, there is hypotension despite adequate fluid replacement, and the need for inotropic or vasopressor support. Multiple-Organ Dysfunction Syndrome (MODS): Altered organ function than cannot maintain homeostasis without intervention.

It is now known that sepsis is more than just the body's response to an infection. Sepsis is a process that includes a multitude of interrelated processes of inflammation and coagulation. Many different hormones and elements work either together or against each other in an attempt to restore the body to a healthy state. Medical research is discovering more and more every day about this complicated life-threatening syndrome.

References

1.   Neviere, Remi. (2010). *Pathophysiology of Sepsis.* Retrieved from http://www.uptodate.com/contents/pathophysiology-of-sepsis
2.   Picard, Kathy M., O'Donoghue, Sharon C., Young-Kershaw, Duane A., and Russell, Kristin J. (2006, June). Development and Implementation of a Multidisciplinary Sepsis Protocol. *Critical Care Nurse*, 26(3) 43-54. Retrieved from http://www.aacn.org/wd/cetests/media/c0633.pdf

CHAPTER 7

Signs and Symptoms of Sepsis

SEPSIS BEGINS WITH AN INFECTION. As we've seen, the immune system reacts to the pathogen by sending potent cellular mediators to the area to eradicate the invading organism. As numerous proteins and cytokines release their chemical messengers, widespread inflammation can occur. The systemic inflammatory response syndrome that follows has a routine and expected list of physical symptoms and clinical laboratory results that coincide with it:

Hypotension—Hypotension from the increased endothelial permeability and reduced arterial tone is the most severe expression of the circulatory dysfunction in sepsis; however, each organ system is affected by the altered circulation.

Body temperature—In the first 6–72 hours of shock, a patient will be in a hyperdynamic warm phase. Phagocytic leukocytes produce pyrogens that stimulate the hypothalamus to generate more heat, resulting in an elevated temperature. As the hypotension and hypoperfusion of sepsis continues, the worsening and often irreversible cold phase of shock begins, resulting in subnormal temperatures.

There are different features of warm and cold stages of shock, as evidenced by the following symptoms:

Warm Shock

- Bounding pulses
- Tachycardia
- Relatively stable blood pressure
- Warm, flushed peripheries
- <2-second capillary refill
- Widened pulse pressure

Cold Shock

- Weak pulses
- Tachycardia or bradycardia
- Hypotension
- Cold, clammy skin
- >2-second capillary refill
- Narrowed pulse pressure

Neurological—Impaired microcirculation in the brain and other organs is caused by the vasoconstriction from the production of cytokines, interferons, and interleukins. The result is decreased level of consciousness, and confusion.

Circulation—The increased vascular permeability from cytokine production causes hypovolemia and decreased cardiac output. Heart rate increases as the body tries to compensate for the decreased volume (shock). Other signs of impaired circulation can include skin mottling or cyanosis.

Respiratory—One of the earliest signs of sepsis can be an elevated respiratory rate from hypoxemia. This is due to the cytokine-mediated effects on the respiratory center that causes pulmonary edema secondary to capillary leak, or shunting of deoxygenated blood through the lungs. Disturbed capillary blood flow along with endothelial injury in the pulmonary vasculature leads to the formation of pulmonary edema. Arterial hypoxemia and ventilation-perfusion mismatch contribute further to the acute respiratory distress syndrome (ARDS) that often accompanies sepsis.

Kidneys—Hypotension, cytokine activity, and direct renal vasoconstriction contribute to the formation of acute tubular necrosis that often accompanies sepsis. Worsening renal function as well as low urine output, electrolyte imbalances, and anuria (oliguria in the early phases) occurs.

Gastrointestinal tract— When a patient is on the ventilator and is not eating, the overgrowth of bacteria can be aspirated into the lungs, resulting in nosocomial pneumonia. Decreased circulation depresses the stomach's normal barrier functions and allows the translocation of bacteria and other endotoxins that can worsen the sepsis response.

Liver—Poor circulation leads to liver dysfunction. Normally, the reticuloendothelial system of the liver is the first line of defense in clearing the portal system of bacteria that have entered the liver from the gut. Failure of this leads to an inappropriate cytokine response and the possibility of the bacteria-derived products entering the systemic circulation. Signs of liver dysfunction include elevated bilirubin, jaundiced skin, low albumin, and decreased clotting factors.

Nervous system—Symptoms of central nervous system dysfunction include muscle weakness, reduced or absent deep tendon reflexes, and loss of peripheral sensation to light touch. This is due to changes in metabolism and to the inflammatory mediators decreasing the cells' ability to signal each other.

Clinical Signs of Sepsis

Along with the physically visible manifestations of sepsis, chemical changes in the body may manifest, which laboratory tests will display results out of the normal range.

CBC—White blood cells are a major part of the immune system. They are produced in the bone marrow and travel through the blood, searching for infected tissue, where they can ingest bacteria, viruses, parasites, or fungi. There are many types of white blood cells, and each one specializes in a different task. White blood cells are either granulocytes (the presence of granules in the cytoplasm) or agranulocyte lymphoid cells (lacking granules in the cytoplasm).

Granulocytes

- Neutrophils—Present in large amounts in the pus of a wound. They eat invading bacteria. Immature neutrophils are also known as bands. Elevated bands (>10%) are one of the first signs of sepsis. They are produced in response to an infection; an elevation in bands is called a shift to the left.
- Eosinophils—Attack parasites.
- Basophils—Secrete anticoagulant and vasodilatory substances to mediate a hypersensitivity reaction.

Agranulocytes (Lymphoid Cells)

- Lymphocytes—Circulate mostly in a resting state. Lymphocytes carry antibodies that recognize antigens and attach to them.
- Monocytes—Migrate to areas of infection to work as phagocytes (engulf and digest invading organisms).

The number of white blood cells (WBCs) normally ranges from 4,500 to 10,000 per microliter (mcL) of blood, depending on the sex and size of the individual. (Be aware that all ranges can vary slightly from lab to lab.) Elevated WBCs (>30,000) can indicate a systemic inflammatory response such as with sepsis or in a tissue injury from burns and trauma. Other factors that can elevate WBC count include stress, smoking, leukemia, or certain medications such as antibiotics or seizure drugs.

In the later stages of sepsis, WBC count may be low because of the body's inability to keep up with the demand.

Lactic acid—Lactate is a milk acid that is produced by the body to provide energy. It is a major component of the complex process of glycolysis, in which the glycogen in the muscles breaks down into glucose, splits into two pyruvic acid molecules, and releases energy known as adenosine triphosphate (ATP). Normally, the pyruvic acid will merge with the mitochondria, forming more ATP via the oxidation process. This is especially useful during times of exercise.

During sepsis, however, or when there is hypoxemia and poor circulation, the result is poor energy production by the mitochondria because the oxygen is not available. In this case, the pyruvic acid is transformed into lactic acid.

The lactic acid levels accumulate faster than the liver can break them down, resulting in lactic acidosis.

A normal lactate level is <2 mmol/L. In a mildly elevated condition, lactate levels can range from 2 to 5 mmol/L. Levels >4 mmol/L are associated with metabolic acidosis.

C-reactive protein (CRP)—CRP is a protein produced in response to infection, inflammation, or some kind of tissue injury. It is used to assess the status of bacterial infections and chronic inflammation. It is also used to evaluate the response to current therapy. The levels of CRP rise within 2–3 days of an acute stimulus, then fall over 1–2 weeks as the infection clears and/or inflammation subsides. Normal levels should be approximately 2–4.9 mg/L.

Procalcitonin (PCT) is a precursor to the hormone calcitonin. Normally, PCT is converted to calcitonin and stays in the thyroid, but the various cytokines that are released in sepsis prevent the conversion from completing. This results in very high levels of PCT in the blood. Normal levels should be <0.5 ng/ml.

An astute and well-educated nurse will be able to recognize these warning signs of sepsis and initiate appropriate treatment in a timely manner.

In review, the signs and symptoms to be alert for are listed below. (Sepsis Symptoms, 2012).

General

- Fever
- Hypothermia
- Heart rate >90 bpm
- Fast respiratory rate

- Altered mental status (confusion/coma)
- Edema (swelling)
- High blood glucose without diabetes

Inflammatory

- High WBC count
- Low WBC count
- Immature WBCs in the circulation
- Elevated plasma C-reactive protein
- Elevated PCT

Hemodynamic

- Low blood pressure
- Low central venous or mixed venous oxygen saturation
- High cardiac index

Organ Dysfunction

- Low oxygen level
- Low urine output
- High creatinine
- Coagulation abnormalities
- Absent bowel sounds
- Low platelets
- High bilirubin

Tissue Perfusion

- High lactate
- Decreased capillary filling or mottling

Reference

1.   Sepsis Alliance. (2012). Sepsis Symptoms. Retrieved from http://www.sepsisalliance.org/sepsis/symptoms/

CHAPTER 8

Sepsis Treatment

IN 2002, THE EUROPEAN SOCIETY of Critical Care Medicine and the Society of Critical Care Medicine (SCCM) conducted an international survey of physicians' views of sepsis. The results verified that sepsis is a challenging and frustrating syndrome that is often misattributed to other conditions and that physicians are eager for a breakthrough in the treatment regime. Many physicians also agreed that a common definition for sepsis in the medical community would be a beneficial step in the right direction.

The Surviving Sepsis Campaign was spearheaded by the ESICM (European Society of Intensive Care Medicine), the ISF (International Sepsis Forum), and the SCCM with a goal of improving the diagnosis, survival, and management of patients with sepsis. (For further information, please visit the Surviving Sepsis Campaign web site at http://www.survivingsepsis.org/Pages/default.aspx)

The treatment bundles discussed in this chapter are adapted with permission (Copyright 2008, European Society of Intensive Care Medicine and Society of Critical Care Medicine).

By the time this book publishes, the ESICM and the SCCM, with input from the Institute for Healthcare Improvement, will have updated recommendations and changed the treatment bundles, affecting the accuracy of the guidelines poster and some of the content of this chapter. Please visit www.survivingsepsiscampaign.org for the updated recommendations.

Bundles

A bundle is a group of therapies for a certain disease process (or syndrome, in this case) that, when implemented together, can substantially improve patient outcomes. Each element comes from evidence-based practices and has been designed to achieve a 25% reduction in mortality from severe sepsis or septic shock.

These custom-created therapies should be used as a guide, a pathway for each hospital to institute into its own protocols. There are two severe sepsis bundles. The first bundle, "sepsis resuscitation," includes 7 tasks (in 5 bundle groups) that should be implemented as soon as severe sepsis has been identified. The goal is to implement each element within 6 hours of identification 100% of the time.

The second bundle, "sepsis management," includes 3 tasks (one in each bundle group), that should be completed within 24 hours for patients with severe sepsis, septic shock, and/or lactate >4 mmol/L. Some of the elements of the bundle may be omitted, depending on the clinical conditions if the patient does not meet the parameters for giving the treatment. The goal here is to perform all indicated tasks within 24 hours of presentation 100% of the time.

Not every institution has developed a sepsis protocol as of yet. Check the policy and procedures where you work to see if a policy has been enacted. Even if one hasn't been, you can still understand the process and encourage physicians to comply with the bundle therapies.

Sepsis Resuscitation Bundle

Bundle Element 1—Measure Serum Lactate

Elevated serum lactate levels (hyperlactatemia) are due to anaerobic metabolism secondary to hypoperfusion. Although hyperlactatemia can be due to other conditions such as decreased clearance by the liver, it is essential to obtain a serum lactate level to identify tissue hypoperfusion for patients who may not yet be showing signs of hypotension. The prognostic value of elevated lactate levels has been well established and holds greater value than oxygen-derived variables.

- Regardless of blood pressure, if a serum lactate level is >4 mmol/L, begin the sepsis resuscitation bundle.

It is very important that your institution has a quick turnaround time so that the lactate level may be received from the lab within minutes. Receiving lab results from a typical venipuncture specimen may take 24–48 hours and this is unacceptable. It has been recommended by some researchers that all institutions invest in the appropriate equipment, such as blood gas analyzers, that use arterial blood to obtain rapid results. The other benefit to using arterial blood is that no tourniquet is required that may hinder clinical care.

Bundle Element 2—Obtain Blood Cultures Prior to Administering Antibiotics

Thirty to fifty percent (30%–50%) of patients with severe sepsis or shock have positive blood cultures. Administering an antibiotic without checking blood cultures first, could prevent the blood culture from adequately revealing the presence of blood-borne pathogens. Two or more blood cultures are recommended to be drawn at the same time from different sites.

If a catheter-related infection is suspected, blood should be drawn from the catheter hub at the same time a peripheral sample is drawn. If the same organism is present in both samples, it can be inferred that the organism in the cultures is the source of infection. Also, if the blood drawn from the catheter hub is positive much earlier than the blood obtained by a peripheral stick, it may also be inferred that the catheter is the source of the infection.

Bundle Element 3—Improve Time to Broad-Spectrum Antibiotics

Antibiotics must be started as soon as possible after sepsis has been identified. The duration of hypotension prior to the administration of antibiotics has been proven to be a major factor in the patient's chance for survival. In a recent study of patients with ventilator-acquired pneumonia (VAP), it was found that patients with significant organ dysfunction who received antibiotics later had a significant increase in mortality: 37% versus 7% in ICU and 44% versus 15% in the hospital.

From the time of presentation, broad-spectrum antibiotics should be administered within 3 hours for emergency department admissions and within 1 hour for non-emergency department ICU admissions.

The major causes of severe sepsis or septic shock are pneumonia and intra-abdominal infections (the other sources account for less than 5% of severe sepsis); however, the true cause of severe sepsis in a patient will be unknown until blood, sputum, and/or urine cultures are collected, which is problematic because it can take 2–3 days to get the results of these cultures.

Because antibiotic therapy cannot wait for the cultures to be completed, broad-spectrum antibiotics should be given until the causative agent of the sepsis has been identified. When the causative agent has been identified, usually 48–72 hours later, the appropriate antibiotic can be initiated and the number of antibiotics given can be restricted to narrow the spectrum of antimicrobial therapy. This will not only reduce costs but also prevent the development of resistance and reduce toxicity.

All patients should receive a full loading dose of each antimicrobial but, because of hepatic or renal function, some may need the concentrations adjusted by the ICU pharmacist. The duration of typical therapy runs for approximately 7–10 days and is guided by the clinical response.

- Infuse antibiotics through multiple lines as available in order to speed delivery of agents.

It is important to remember to cover both gram-positive and gram-negative organisms, as well as to consider double antibiotics for pseudomonas if the clinical situation warrants. Remember also to consider specific knowledge about the patient's history and what he or she may have been exposed to.

Bundle Element 4—Treat Hypotension and/or Elevated Lactate with Fluids

Patients who have hypotension and/or have a lactate level >4 mmol/L are at great risk of vasodilation and impaired cardiac output. These patients must be treated with intravenous fluids to expand the circulating volume and to restore perfusion pressure.

An initial fluid challenge should be given as soon as possible of either:

- Crystalloid—20ml/kg (isotonic solutions such as normal saline or lactated ringers)
- Colloid—0.2g/kg – 0.3 g/kg, depending on type

Clinical studies comparing crystalloid and colloid therapies indicate that there is no difference in the outcome of either albumin or normal saline. The important thing to remember is that crystalloid therapy requires larger doses than colloid therapy and results in more edema.

Patients who are receiving fluid challenge, regardless of type, need to be closely monitored and require the definition of four components:

1. The type of fluid to be administered (i.e., normal saline, albumin, blood products, etc.)
2. The rate of the infusion (typically ranges from 500 to 1000 cc over 30 minutes)
3. The endpoints to monitor [such as mean arterial pressure (MAP) >70 or heart rate <110 bpm)

4.   Safety limits (such as pulmonary and/or systemic edema)

After the fluid challenge is completed, the maintenance dose is generally increased, and, because of venodilation and capillary leak, additional fluid challenges may be required to avoid hypotension for the first 24 hours of the sepsis resuscitation.

It is recommended for the initial fluid challenge to target a CVP of at least 8mm Hg, or 12 mm Hg in mechanically ventilated patients.

If the patient's blood pressure is not responding to the fluid challenge, consider other causes of low blood pressure, such as depressed myocardial function, adrenal insufficiency, tension pneumothorax, cardiac tamponade, and the like.

Apply vasopressors for ongoing hypotension. In the event that a fluid challenge does not improve hypotension to a mean arterial pressure of at least 65 mm Hg, therapy with vasopressor agents should be started. Remember, however, that adequate fluid resuscitation is a prerequisite for successful vasopressor therapy. Remain watchful for these potential detrimental effects of vasopressors:

• Worsening inadequate organ perfusion (from the vasoconstriction), especially if the patient is inadequately volume resuscitated; the patient may simply need more fluids.
• Worsening cardiac output from the increased left ventricular workload, especially in patients with preexisting heart disease.

The variety of vasopressors to choose from includes epinephrine, phenylephrine (Neo-Synephrine), dopamine, norepinephrine (Levophed), and vasopressin. Each drug has its own set of risks and precautions to consider.

Epinephrine— Not considered a first-line drug of choice in the treatment of sepsis. It decreases splanchnic blood flow, increases gastric mucosal pCO2 production, and decreases PH.

Phenylephrine (Neo-Synephrine)— Also not considered a first-line drug of choice in the treatment of sepsis because it decreases splanchnic blood flow and oxygen delivery in patients with septic shock.

Vasopressin—May be considered for patients with refractory shock despite adequate fluid resuscitation and high-dose vasopressors. Not recommended as a replacement for norepinephrine or dopamine as a first-line agent until the results of ongoing trials are reviewed. (.03 units/minute of vasopressin may be subsequently added to norepinephrine with anticipation of an effect equivalent to norepinephrine alone.)

Dopamine—Increases heart rate, systemic vascular resistance (SVR), and stroke volume to increase cardiac index (CI). Dopamine also alters the inflammatory response in septic shock by decreasing the release of certain hormones such as prolactin. Dopamine's effect on the gastric mucosa is unclear, and it may have other harmful side effects in patients with septic shock.

Norepinephrine (Levophed)—Increases mean arterial pressure (MAP) secondary to vasoconstriction and does not affect heart rate or cardiac output (CO). Historically, it was believed that norepinephrine had negative effects on blood flow in the splanchnic and renal vascular beds that resulted in regional ischemia and was used only as a last-resort medication, often with poor results. It is now known that norepinephrine both provides vascular tone and makes minor improvements in contractility (90% alpha, 10% beta). Norepinephrine often does not cause the profound tachycardia that dopamine does; therefore, in septic shock, when the vascular tone is lost and the patient has profound vasodilation, norepinephrine is the perfect drug of choice. Best outcomes occur when norepinephrine is titrated appropriately.

The Surviving Sepsis Campaign advises using either norepinephrine or dopamine as a first-line drug of choice for low blood pressure in patients with septic shock. Epinephrine should be a second-line drug of choice if norepinephrine or dopamine are not effective.

The objective of fluid treatment is to maintain a mean arterial blood pressure of at least 65. This will ensure that all internal organs are being perfused adequately. Sometimes the fluid challenge alone may achieve this; however, it is often necessary to add appropriate vasopressor therapy. The following are points to remember:

1. The patient must be transferred to an ICU for appropriate treatment.
2. Insertion of an arterial line is necessary for the continuous monitoring of blood pressure.
3. Potential detrimental effects may occur if vasopressor therapy is initiated prior to adequate fluid resuscitation. Conversely, therapy should not be delayed if the blood pressure is severely low.
4. The use of vasopressors remains controversial, as they raise the blood pressure at the expense of internal organs such as kidneys and stomach.

5. Controversy exists as to whether the overenthusiastic use of vasopressors targets an unnecessarily high blood pressure that results in increased left ventricular workload, thereby worsening cardiac output and end-organ perfusion.

Bundle Element 5—Maintain Adequate Central Venous Pressure (CVP) and Adequate Central Venous Oxygen Saturation (ScVO2)

According to the Surviving Sepsis Campaign, "Once lactate is >4 mmol/L, or hypotension has been demonstrated to be refractive to an initial fluid challenge with 20 mL/kg of crystalloid or colloid equivalent, patients should have their CVP maintained >8 mm Hg and central venous oxygen saturation should be maintained >70 percent."

Due to the presence of increased intrathoracic pressure from the positive end expiratory pressure in mechanically ventilated patients, it is recommended that their CVP be kept at 12–15 mm Hg.

If a patient both is hypovolemic and has a low hematocrit (<30%), it would be prudent to consider the infusion of red blood cells, provided that the fluid challenge has brought the CVP up to at least 8 mm Hg. If the CVP is not at least 8, additional fluid challenges are needed.

Infusing blood will not only help to elevate the CVP and keep it up but will also improve the ScVO2 by increasing oxygen delivery to the tissue beds.

If the cardiac output remains low despite adequate circulating volume, it may be necessary to add an inotropic medication such as dobutamine.

Continuous ScVO2 can reveal early tissue hypoxia before it is reflected in the vital signs. It is a more sensitive indicator of tissue perfusion compared to traditional vital-sign monitoring or intermittent sampling. ScVO2 is monitored with the placement of a central venous catheter equipped with a fiber-optic sensor or by numerous repeated blood samples from a traditional catheter.

ScVO2 measures the difference between oxygen consumption and delivery. The normal range for ScVO2 should be around 70%. Lower levels indicate an increased oxygen demand with decreased oxygen delivery, which can be caused by anemia, shivering, suctioning, and the like. Higher levels for ScVO2 indicate that tissues are not using the oxygen that is being delivered (for instance, in a chemically paralyzed patient who is not moving at all).

To help clinicians at the bedside resuscitate patients in septic shock, goal-directed therapy attempts to balance oxygen delivery with demand by adjusting cardiac preload, afterload, and contractility. Two principle strategies are suggested to maintain adequate ScVO2 levels. The first is with packed red blood cell transfusion, as mentioned for CVP monitoring, and the second is with inotropic medications.

For hypotensive patients with lactate levels >4 mmol/L and who have not responded to fluid resuscitation, ScVO2 should be maintained at 70% or greater to reproduce the mortality reductions cited in the literature.

The Surviving Sepsis Campaign states that "Compliance with this sepsis resuscitation bundle element is defined as the percent of patients following septic shock or lactate >4 mmol/L, identification for whom the ScVO2 is >/= 70 percent (or ScVO2 is >/=65 percent) within 6 hours of presentation time."

Sepsis Management Bundle

The second set of bundle therapies must be completed within 24 hours for patients with severe sepsis, septic shock, and/or lactate >4 mmol/L. As many as 4 of these elements must be completed within the first 24 hours for patients with severe sepsis. Depending on the clinical presentation, not all items may need to be completed. It is necessary, however, for clinicians to evaluate for each of the symptoms. The goal is to perform all indicated tasks 100% of the time within the first 24 hours of presentation.

Bundle Element 1—Administer Low-Dose Steroids for Septic Shock in Accordance with a Standardized ICU Policy

For the adult patient in septic shock, when blood pressure is poorly responsive to fluid resuscitation and vasopressor therapy, beginning intravenous corticosteroids is recommended. The usual dose is 200–300 mg/day for seven days in 3 or 4 divided doses, or by continuous infusion. High doses of glucocorticoid therapy for septic shock refers to 30 mg/kg methylprednisolone or equivalent steroid preparations given up to 4 times during a short course of 1 or 2 days; 200–300 mg of hydrocortisone or equivalent may be given daily for 5–7 days or longer for low-dose glucocorticoid trials.

Rapid shock reversal for patients receiving low-dose corticosteroids has been confirmed with numerous randomized controlled trials. Hydrocortisone has been suggested as the preferred glucocorticoid for the following reasons:

1. It is the drug that has been used most for treatment of septic shock.
2. It is the synthetic equivalent to the final active cortisol.
3. It has intrinsic mineralocorticoid activity.

The Surviving Sepsis campaign makes these suggestions regarding the use of steroids:

- Until a policy is in effect in your institution, use the interim low-dose glucocorticoid policy provided in this text.
- To eliminate variation in care, an ICU protocol should be in effect to standardize the use of low-dose steroids.
- Give steroids only to adult patients in septic shock after blood pressure has been identified to be poorly responsive to fluid resuscitation and vasopressor therapy, but don't defer use out of fear of worsening infection.
- Do not use the adrenalcorticotropic hormone (ACTH) stimulation test to identify those who should receive hydrocortisone therapy, as overall trial populations appear to benefit regardless of ACTH test results.
- Do not give dexamethasone to patients in septic shock if hydrocortisone is available.
- Add a daily dose of fludrocortisone 50µg if hydrocortisone is not available and the chosen steroid has no mineralocorticoid activity.
- Wean the patient from steroid therapy when vasopressors are no longer required.
- Use a sufficient dose such as hydrocortisone 50 mg intravenously every 6 hours
- Do not use doses >300 mg daily in severe sepsis or for treating septic shock, as the high-dose therapy is ineffective or harmful, according to studies.
- Do not use corticosteroids in the absence of septic shock.

Bundle Element 2—Maintain Glucose Control Lower Limit of Normal but <180 mg/dL

Effectively maintaining glucose control in the ICU has been shown to decrease mortality and morbidity across a large range of conditions. Patients who have received intensive insulin therapy are less likely to require prolonged mechanical ventilation, and the number of deaths from multiple organ failure with sepsis was also reduced, regardless of patients' history of diabetes or hyperglycemia. Insulin therapy has also halved the prevalence of the following:

- Transfusion requirement
- Prolonged inflammation
- Acute renal failure (ARF) requiring dialysis or hemofiltration
- Bloodstream infections
- Critical illness polyneuropathy

If blood glucose monitoring has not already been ordered, the bedside nurse needs to contact the physician to get it started.

Bundle Element 3—Maintain a Median Inspiratory Plateau Pressure (IPP) <30 cm H2O for mechanically ventilated patients

Most patients with severe sepsis and septic shock will require endotracheal intubation and mechanical ventilation, as they are at increased risk of developing acute lung injury (ALI) or acute respiratory distress syndrome (ARDS). Clinical evidence of lung injury includes

- bilateral patchy infiltrates on chest x-ray;

- low PaO2/FiO2 ratios (<300 for ALI or <200 for ARDS); and
- pulmonary capillary wedge pressure <18 cm H2O (measurable only if patient has a Swan-Ganz catheter).

ALI and ARDS cause stiff, noncompliant lungs that result in decreased compliance, ventilation/perfusion mismatch, and shunting. This occurs when the alveolar ventilation does not match the pulmonary capillary blood flow because the blood that passes through the alveoli does not get oxygenated. The deoxygenated circulating blood causes ineffective ventilation which is often referred to as shunting. The shunting causes hypercapnia (elevated PCO2), which is usually avoided but may be permissible in these cases to minimize plateau pressures and tidal volumes. In most instances, an acutely elevated PCO2 causes vasodilation, increased heart rate, increased blood pressure, and increased cardiac output, but to limit increased tidal volumes and minute ventilation, modest hypercapnia is allowed. Hypercapnia is contraindicated in patients with preexisting respiratory acidosis or with increased intracranial pressures because it may worsen both conditions.

Ventilator Management

- Positive end expiratory end pressure (PEEP) is used to prevent lung collapse at the end of exhalation. It also allows using lower amounts of oxygen to prevent potentially toxic levels.
- In the acute phase of illness, avoid synchronized intermittent mandatory ventilation (SIMV) and use mandatory modes of ventilation such as assist control (ACV) or pressure control (PCV) to prevent spontaneously large tidal volumes.

- Tidal volumes should be <6 mL/kg ideal body weight (IBW) to maintain plateau pressures ≤30 cm H2O.
- Monitor plateau pressures rather than tidal volumes to govern ventilator management.
- Slightly elevated PCO2 levels are acceptable as long as the PH is >7.21, unless stated otherwise by the physician, as some may go as low as 7.10.
- Be advised that a sodium bicarbonate drip may be ordered to facilitate the use of permissive hypercapnia.

References

1. Surviving Sepsis Campaign. (n.d.). Maintain adequate central venous oxygen saturation. Retrieved from
http://www.survivingsepsis.org/Pages/default.aspx

Conclusion

ARCHEOLOGISTS HAVE FOUND EVIDENCE OF mankind's battle with sepsis dating back thousands of years. Studies of unearthed human remains verify sepsis as the cause of death in numerous cases all over the world. Ancient scholars such as Homer and Hippocrates describe the treatment of sepsis in a variety of medical records including ancient Egyptian papyrus and various Sanskrit documents.

What may start out as a simple cut, scrape, or communicable disease can quickly progress to an irreversible inflammatory process that affects every organ in the body. Hypotension and vasoconstriction limit perfusion to the vital organs and eventually contribute to multiple-organ dysfunction syndrome. Treatment must begin as soon as possible, and it must include certain therapies that have been discussed in this book here.

Sepsis affects 750,000 people each year, and the additional cost to our nation's healthcare bill from sepsis is estimated around $20 billion. It's impossible to estimate the amount of suffering sepsis that has caused us, but thanks to research and clinical studies, we have come far in our battle with sepsis. To understand its history, causes, risks, and prevention gives us more ammunition to fight with.

This book was written for nurses. It is written for the bedside nurses so they may learn to recognize the early symptoms of sepsis and realize the importance of beginning treatment as soon as possible. Whatever the time, day or night, a nurse will be the first to take action and begin initiating the sepsis bundle therapies.

Winning the Fight against Sepsis:
What Every Nurse Should Know

Questions

1. What is the most severe expression of circulatory dysfunction in sepsis?
   A. Confusion
   B. Fever
   C. Hypotension
   D. Bounding pulses

2. Elevated temperature from the hyperdynamic warm phase of shock occurs in
   A. The first 6–72 hours.
   B. 2 days.
   C. 12 hours.
   D. 12–36 hours.

3. Symptoms of the warm phase of shock include
   A. bounding pulses with tachycardia.
   B. stable blood pressure with a widened pulse pressure.
   C. warm, flushed peripheries with <2-second capillary refill.
   D. all of the above.

4. Skin mottling, cyanosis, and elevated heart rate are symptoms of
   A. renal failure.
   B. cold stage of shock.
   C. impaired circulation.
   D. pneumonia.

5. A form of white blood cell that is produced in response to an infection and that, when elevated, is known as a shift to the left is
   A. basophil.
   B. eosinophil.
   C. monocyte.
   D. neutrophil.

6. Lactic acid is
   A. a milk acid.
   B. produced by the body to provide energy.
   C. elevated in sepsis.
   D. all of the above.

7. The normal level of lactic acid is
   A. >5 mmol/L.
   B. <2 mmol/L.
   C. 2–10 mmol/L.
   D. 4–10 mmol/L.

8. C-reactive protein is produced in response to
   A. an infection.
   B. inflammation.
   C. any kind of tissue injury.
   D. all of the above.

9. Signs and symptoms of sepsis include
    A. fever and altered mental status.
    B. elevated white blood cells and elevated heart rate.
    C. low urine output and low blood pressure.
    D. all of the above.

10. Treatment bundles are a group of therapies for certain disease processes that, when grouped together, can substantially improve patient outcomes.
    A. True
    B. False

11. An elevated serum lactate level indicates
    A. hypertension.
    B. renal failure.
    C. anaerobic metabolism secondary to hypoperfusion.
    D. lactose intolerance.

12. Blood cultures should be obtained
    A. in the morning.
    B. from central IV access only.
    C. prior to beginning antibiotics.
    D. any time the patient's temperature exceeds 101 degrees.

13. What is the proper time frame for patients to receive antibiotics from the time of presentation?
    A. within 4 hours on all admissions
    B. within 2 hours for emergency department admissions, and within 3 hours for ICU admissions
    C. There is no time limit.
    D. within 3 hours for emergency room admissions, and within 1 hour for non-emergency ICU admissions

14. Patients with lactate levels >4 mmol/L and/or with hypotension should be treated with
    A. IV fluids.
    B. vasopressors.
    C. blood transfusion.
    D. antibiotics.

15. For patients receiving IV fluid bolus, the following should be monitored closely:
    A. Temperature, edema, and heart rate
    B. The type of fluid, the rate of infusion, pulmonary or systemic edema, and end points such as mean arterial pressure (MAP) >70, and heart rate <110
    C. Blood pressure and electrolytes
    D. Urine output, respiratory rate, and neurological changes

16. If the fluid challenge does not help the blood pressure, what should be done?
    A. Give another fluid challenge with D51/2 normal saline
    B. Start nitroglycerin drip to decrease oxygen consumption
    C. Give a diuretic
    D. Consider other causes such as depressed myocardial function, adrenal insufficiency, pneumothorax, and so on.

17. Which of the following does the Surviving Sepsis Campaign consider first-line drugs of choice for low blood pressure in patients in septic shock?
    A. Norepinephrine and dopamine
    B. Vasopressin and dopamine
    C. Dopamine and epinephrine
    D. Vasopressin and Levophed

18. Which of the following is true concerning vasopressor therapy in the septic patient?
    A. The mean arterial pressure (MAP) should be at least 50 in order to perfuse all the internal organs.
    B. Vasopressors can be started at any time without regard to the patient's fluid status.
    C. The patient must be transferred to an ICU for arterial line blood pressure monitoring.
    D. Vasopressors only affect blood pressure; they have no effect on the patient's kidneys or gut.

19. If the central venous pressure (CVP) is low, the addition of packed red blood cells is appropriate if the hematocrit is <30% and the MAP remains <65 mg Hg, followed by further fluid challenges to keep CVP >8 mm Hg.
    A. True
    B. False

20. ScVO2 measures
    A. the difference in mean arterial pressure with systolic blood pressure.
    B. the amount of circulating oxygen in the arterial circulation.
    C. the level of oxygen saturating hemoglobin molecules.
    D. the difference between oxygen consumption and oxygen delivery.

21. Sepsis resuscitation bundles are different than sepsis management bundles.
    A. True
    B. False

22. The sepsis management bundle includes 4 elements and must be completed within 24 hours for the patient with
   A.   lactate level <4 mmol/L.
   B.   sepsis.
   C.   severe sepsis or septic shock.
   D.   low blood pressure.

23. Which of the following is not true regarding low-dose steroid therapy for the patient with septic shock?
   A.   It is okay to abruptly stop steroid treatment when the patient has improved.
   B.   Rapid shock reversal has been confirmed in patients who received low-dose corticosteroids.
   C.   Corticosteroids should not be used in the absence of septic shock.
   D.   Dexamethasone should not be given to patients in septic shock if hydrocortisone is available

24. Blood glucose levels should be maintained below 180 mg/dL because
   A.   higher blood glucose levels decrease infections.
   B.   mechanical ventilation requirements are lower with blood glucose >180.
   C.   fewer deaths occur when blood glucose is kept >180 mg/dl.
   D.   mortality and morbidity are decreased with effective blood glucose management.

25. Which of the following is true regarding mechanical ventilation in the septic patient?

    A. Median inspiratory plateau pressure (IPP) should be maintained <30 cm H2O.

    B. Acute lung injury (ACI) or adult respiratory distress syndrome (ARDS) causes stiff, noncompliant lungs.

    C. Positive end expiratory pressure (PEEP) is used to prevent lung collapse at the end of exhalation.

    D. All of the above are true.

Answer Sheet

1. C
2. A
3. D
4. C
5. D
6. D
7. B
8. D
9. D
10. A
11. C
12. C
13. D
14. A
15. B
16. D
17. A
18. C
19. A
20. D
21. A
22. C
23. A
24. D
25. D

AUTHOR BIOGRAPHY

Melissa was born in Cheverly, Maryland, in 1965 and had many different homes as her family moved frequently. She spent the majority of her childhood on a farm in Michigan where she enjoyed her horses and gardening. She moved to Florida in 1983 and worked various small jobs before she became a nurse. She worked as a receptionist in a veterinarian's office, a law office, and in a bond-brokerage firm; she also worked as a certified nurse's aide, co-managed an RV park, and worked on a thoroughbred horse farm with her husband, Bill. She finally decided that she wanted a real career and enrolled in nursing school in 1987. She graduated in 1990 and has spent the past 22 years working mostly on weekend night shifts in ICU. She achieved CCRN certification in 2001 and earned her bachelor's degree in nursing from Florida State University in 2005.

Her goal now is to write not only educational and informative books for nurses but also to expand her fiction-writing skills.

The Traveler: In the Beginning (available from Dog Ear Publishing, Amazon, and Barnes and Noble) is the first book in her series written for anyone with an interest in the paranormal.

Lightning Source UK Ltd.
Milton Keynes UK
UKOW06f1921010915

257918UK00018B/563/P